Fatty Liver Diet Cookbook for Seniors

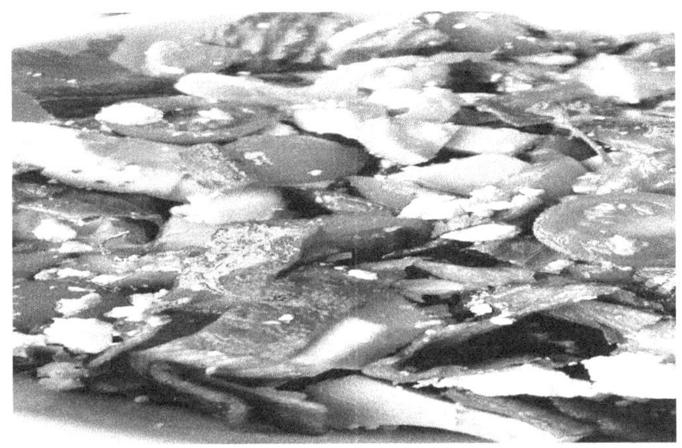

A Comprehensive Guide to Nourishing Your Liver and Embracing Wellness in Your Golden Years

Isaac Hendricks

Table Of Contents

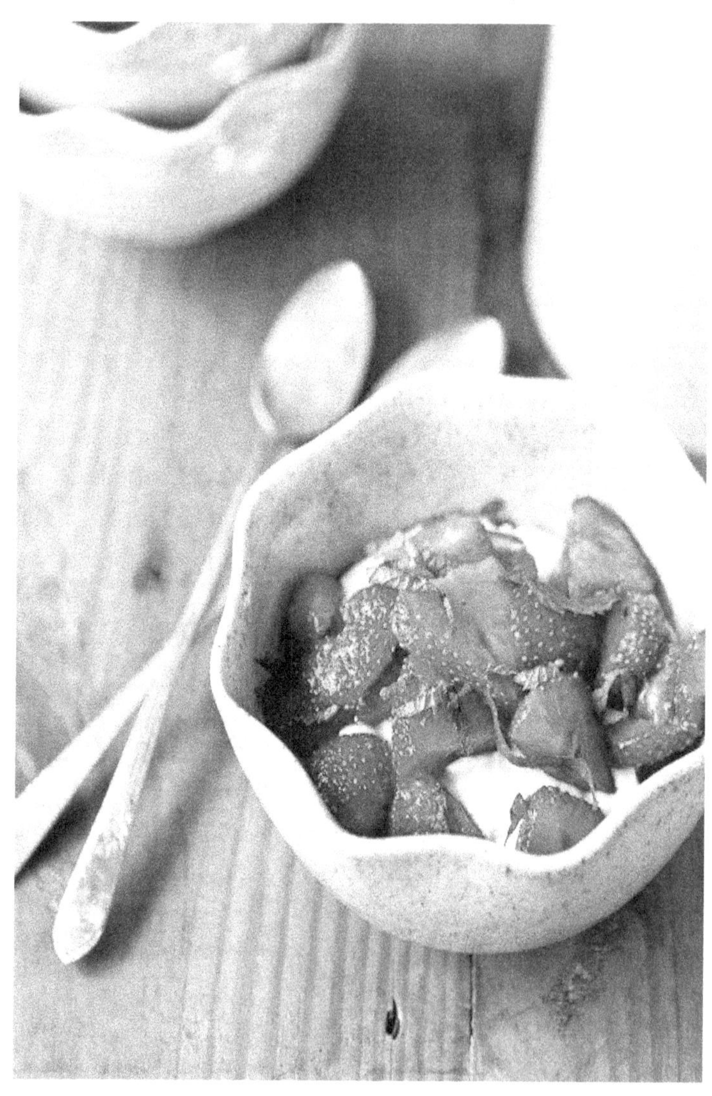

INTRODUCTION

Welcome to the "Fatty Liver Diet Cookbook for Seniors." This comprehensive guide is tailored specifically for seniors who are grappling with the challenges of managing fatty liver disease. Fatty liver disease is a common condition characterised by the accumulation of fat in the liver cells. It's a growing concern among seniors, often attributed to lifestyle factors, diet, and age-related changes in metabolism.

As we gracefully navigate the golden years, our bodies, like seasoned voyagers, require special attention and care. Among the myriad health concerns that often accompany ageing, the spectre of fatty liver disease looms large. Yet, fear not, for within these pages lies a treasure trove of culinary wisdom, meticulously crafted to support liver health and overall well-being.

In this cookbook, we aim to provide seniors with practical strategies and delicious recipes to support liver health and overall well-being. Our approach emphasises the importance of nutrition, mindful eating, and lifestyle modifications in managing fatty liver disease effectively.

Fatty liver disease can lead to serious complications if left untreated, including liver inflammation, scarring (cirrhosis), and even liver failure. However, with the right diet and lifestyle changes, seniors can significantly improve liver function and mitigate the progression of the disease.

Throughout this book, we'll delve into the fundamentals of fatty liver disease, explore the role of diet in its management, and provide you with a wealth of senior-friendly recipes and meal plans designed to nourish your body and support liver health.

Whether you've recently been diagnosed with fatty liver disease or you're proactively seeking ways to optimise your health, this cookbook is your comprehensive resource for navigating the challenges of managing fatty liver as a senior.

CHAPTER ONE

Understanding Fatty Liver: Causes and Symptoms

Fatty liver disease, also known as hepatic steatosis, arises when fat accumulates in the liver's cells. This condition is typically categorised into two main types: alcoholic fatty liver disease and non-alcoholic fatty liver disease (NAFLD).

Causes of Fatty Liver:

Fatty liver disease, commonly known as hepatic steatosis, can be caused by many reasons, including:

Poor Diet: Consuming high amounts of unhealthy fats, sugars, and processed foods can contribute to the accumulation of fat in the liver.

Obesity: Excessive body weight, especially abdominal obesity, is strongly linked to fatty liver disease. Fat accumulation in the liver is often associated with being overweight or obese.

Insulin Resistance: When cells become resistant to the effects of insulin, the body produces more insulin to compensate. This can lead to increased fat accumulation in the liver.

Type 2 Diabetes: Individuals with type 2 diabetes are at a higher risk of developing fatty liver disease due to insulin resistance and other metabolic factors.

High Blood Lipids: Elevated levels of triglycerides and cholesterol in the blood can contribute to the accumulation of fat in the liver.

Genetics: Some people may inherit genes that predispose them to fatty liver disease, even in the absence of other risk factors.

Alcohol Consumption: Excessive alcohol consumption is a leading cause of alcoholic fatty liver disease. Alcohol is metabolised in the liver, and heavy drinking can lead to inflammation and fatty deposits.

Medications: Certain medications, including corticosteroids, tamoxifen, methotrexate, and others, can contribute to fat accumulation in the liver.

Rapid Weight Loss: Losing weight too quickly, especially through crash diets or bariatric surgery, can cause the liver to release stored fat, leading to fatty liver disease.

Other Medical Conditions: Conditions such as metabolic syndrome, polycystic ovary syndrome

(PCOS), hypothyroidism, and sleep apnea can increase the risk of fatty liver disease.

Addressing these underlying causes through lifestyle changes, dietary modifications, weight management, and medical interventions can help prevent and manage fatty liver disease.

Symptoms of Fatty Liver:

Fatty liver disease often progresses silently without causing noticeable symptoms in its early stages. However, as the condition advances, some individuals may experience the following symptoms:

1. **Fatigue:** Feeling tired or fatigued even after adequate rest is a common symptom of fatty liver disease. The liver's impaired function can lead to decreased energy levels.

2. **Weakness:** Weakness or a sense of overall malaise may accompany fatigue in individuals with fatty liver disease.

3. **Abdominal Discomfort:** Some people with fatty liver disease may experience discomfort or pain in the upper right side of the abdomen, where the liver is located. This discomfort may be dull and persistent or sharp and intermittent.

4. **Swelling in the Abdomen:** Accumulation of fluid in the abdomen, known as ascites, can occur in advanced stages of fatty liver disease. This can cause abdominal swelling and a feeling of heaviness.

5. **Jaundice:** In some cases, fatty liver disease can lead to jaundice, characterised by yellowing of the skin and the whites of the eyes. Jaundice arises when the liver is unable to handle bilirubin efficiently.

6. **Loss of Appetite:** A decreased desire to eat or a feeling of fullness even after consuming small amounts of food can occur in individuals with fatty liver disease.

7. **Nausea and Vomiting:** Some people may experience nausea, vomiting, or a general feeling of queasiness, especially after consuming fatty or rich foods.

8. **Weakness and Unexplained Weight Loss:** As fatty liver disease progresses, individuals may experience unexplained weight loss and muscle weakness due to the liver's decreased ability to metabolise nutrients.

9. **Dark Urine:** Urine may appear darker than usual due to the presence of bilirubin, a waste product that is not effectively processed by the liver in individuals with fatty liver disease.

10. **<u>Spider Veins and Skin Changes:</u>** Spider veins (small, dilated blood vessels) may appear on the skin, particularly on the upper body, along with other skin changes such as redness or discoloration.

It's important to note that not everyone with fatty liver disease will experience symptoms, and the severity and combination of symptoms can vary widely among individuals. Seeking medical attention and undergoing appropriate diagnostic tests are crucial for identifying and managing fatty liver disease effectively.

Risk Factors for Fatty Liver:

- Obesity and excess body weight
- Type 2 diabetes or insulin resistance
- High blood pressure
- High cholesterol or triglyceride levels
- Sedentary lifestyle
- Poor dietary habits, including consumption of high-fat and high-sugar foods

Understanding these risk factors can help individuals take proactive steps to reduce their risk of developing fatty liver disease. Lifestyle modifications, such as maintaining a healthy weight, following a balanced diet, exercising regularly, limiting alcohol consumption, and managing underlying medical conditions, can help mitigate the risk of fatty liver disease. Regular medical check-ups and screenings are also important for early detection and management of fatty liver disease.

In the following chapters, we'll explore the role of diet, nutrition, and lifestyle modifications in managing fatty liver disease effectively, especially for seniors.

CHAPTER TWO

Importance of Diet in Managing Fatty Liver

Diet plays a pivotal role in the management of fatty liver disease. For seniors, adopting a liver-friendly diet can help alleviate symptoms, reduce inflammation, and improve overall liver function. In this chapter, we'll delve into the key dietary principles for managing fatty liver:

Limiting Saturated and Trans Fats:

- ❖ Saturated and trans fats are known to contribute to liver inflammation and worsen fatty liver disease.

- ❖ Seniors should aim to minimise their intake of foods high in saturated and trans fats, such as red meat, processed foods, fried foods, and baked goods.

Emphasising Healthy Fats:

- ❖ Incorporating healthy fats into the diet, such as those found in avocados, nuts, seeds, and fatty fish like salmon and mackerel, can support liver health and reduce inflammation.

- ❖ Fibre-rich foods, including fruits, vegetables, whole grains, and legumes, can aid in weight management, regulate blood sugar levels, and promote healthy digestion, which is beneficial for individuals with fatty liver disease.

Monitoring Sugar Consumption:

- ❖ Excessive sugar consumption, especially from sugary beverages and processed foods, can contribute to insulin resistance and exacerbate fatty liver disease.

- ❖ Seniors should opt for natural sources of sweetness, such as fresh fruits, and limit their intake of added sugars and refined carbohydrates.

Moderating Alcohol Consumption:

- ❖ For seniors with fatty liver disease, it's crucial to limit or abstain from alcohol consumption altogether, as alcohol can further damage the liver and exacerbate existing liver conditions.

By adopting a balanced and nutritious diet rich in whole foods, seniors can effectively manage fatty liver disease and improve their overall health and well-being.

Role of Nutrition in Liver Health

Nutrition plays a pivotal role in maintaining liver health, particularly for seniors who may be more susceptible to liver issues like fatty liver disease. Here's how dietary choices can positively impact liver function:

1. ***Reducing Fat Intake:*** Seniors should aim to limit saturated and trans fats in their diet. These fats can contribute to the accumulation of fat in the liver, leading to fatty liver disease. Instead, focus on eating healthy fats such as avocados, nuts, seeds, and fatty fish.

2. ***Emphasising Plant-Based Foods:*** A diet rich in fruits, vegetables, whole grains, and legumes provides essential nutrients and antioxidants that support liver health. These foods also contain fibre, which aids in digestion and helps to maintain a healthy weight.

3. ***Moderating Sugar Consumption:*** Excessive sugar intake can lead to insulin resistance and contribute to the development of non-alcoholic fatty liver disease (NAFLD). Seniors should limit their intake of sugary foods and beverages, opting for natural sources of sweetness like fruits instead.

4. ***Watching Sodium Levels:*** High sodium intake can lead to fluid retention and liver damage.

Seniors should be mindful of their sodium intake and opt for low-sodium alternatives when possible.

5. ***Promoting Hydration:*** Staying hydrated is essential for liver health as it helps to flush toxins from the body and supports proper liver function. Seniors should attempt to drink enough of water throughout the day.

6. ***Limiting Alcohol:*** Excessive alcohol consumption can cause liver inflammation and damage over time. Seniors should follow recommended guidelines for alcohol consumption or abstain from alcohol altogether, especially if they have liver-related health concerns.

7. ***Balancing Micronutrients:*** Consuming a balanced diet that includes adequate levels of vitamins and minerals is essential for overall liver health. Nutrients like vitamin E, vitamin C, selenium, and zinc have been shown to support liver function and reduce inflammation.

8. ***Seeking Professional Guidance:*** Seniors with existing liver conditions or concerns should consult with a healthcare provider or a registered dietitian to develop a personalised nutrition plan tailored to their specific needs and medical history.

By adopting a nutritious and liver-friendly diet, seniors can help support liver health and reduce the risk of developing liver-related complications. A well-balanced diet, combined with regular physical activity and healthy lifestyle choices, can contribute to overall well-being and longevity.

Dietary Guidelines for Seniors with Fatty Liver

Seniors diagnosed with fatty liver disease need to adhere to dietary guidelines that can help manage the condition and prevent its progression. Here are some key dietary recommendations tailored for seniors with fatty liver:

1. Limit Saturated and Trans Fats: Seniors should reduce their intake of saturated and trans fats found in fried foods, processed snacks, fatty meats, and baked goods. These fats can exacerbate liver inflammation and contribute to the accumulation of fat in the liver.

2. Focus on Healthy Fats: Instead of saturated and trans fats, seniors should incorporate healthier fat sources into their diet, such as avocados, nuts, seeds, olive oil, and fatty fish like salmon and mackerel. These fats provide essential fatty acids and can help reduce inflammation in the liver.

3. Increase Fibre Intake: Fibre-rich foods like fruits, vegetables, whole grains, and legumes aid in digestion and help regulate

blood sugar levels. They also promote satiety, which can help seniors maintain a healthy weight. Fibre can also help reduce the absorption of fat in the liver, which is beneficial for those with fatty liver disease.

4. Moderate Protein Consumption: Seniors should aim for a moderate intake of lean protein sources such as poultry, fish, tofu, legumes, and low-fat dairy products. Protein is essential for tissue repair and muscle maintenance, but excessive protein intake can strain the liver. Consulting with a healthcare provider or dietitian can help determine the appropriate protein intake for individual needs.

5. Limit Sugar and Refined Carbohydrates: High consumption of sugar and refined carbohydrates can contribute to insulin resistance and worsen fatty liver disease. Seniors should reduce their intake of sugary beverages, sweets, white bread, and pastries, opting instead for whole grain alternatives and naturally sweetened foods like fruits.

6. Monitor Portion Sizes: Controlling portion sizes can help seniors manage their calorie intake and maintain a healthy weight. Overeating can lead to weight gain and increase the risk of fatty liver disease

progression. Using smaller plates, practising mindful eating, and paying attention to hunger and fullness cues can help regulate portion sizes.

7. Stay Hydrated: Adequate hydration is important for liver health as it helps flush toxins from the body and supports overall metabolism. Seniors should aim to drink plenty of water throughout the day, especially in hot weather or during physical activity.

8. Limit Alcohol Consumption: Seniors with fatty liver disease should limit or avoid alcohol consumption altogether. Alcohol can exacerbate liver damage and interfere with liver function, worsening the symptoms of fatty liver disease.

9. Seek Professional Guidance: Seniors with fatty liver disease should work closely with their healthcare provider or a registered dietitian to develop a personalised nutrition plan tailored to their specific needs and medical history. Regular monitoring and adjustments to the diet may be necessary to effectively manage the condition.

By following these dietary guidelines and making healthy lifestyle choices, seniors with fatty liver disease can help improve liver function, reduce inflammation, and prevent complications associated with the condition. Consistency and commitment to a balanced diet and active lifestyle are key to managing fatty liver disease effectively.

CHAPTER THREE

Nutritional Guidelines for Seniors with Fatty Liver

Seniors with fatty liver disease require special attention to their nutritional needs to support liver health and overall vitality. In this chapter, we'll outline practical nutritional guidelines tailored specifically for seniors managing fatty liver disease:

Focus on Whole Foods:

★ Encourage seniors to prioritise whole, minimally processed foods in their diet, including fruits, vegetables, whole grains, lean proteins, and healthy fats.

★ Whole foods provide essential nutrients, antioxidants, and fibre, which are beneficial for liver health and overall well-being.

Stay Hydrated:

★ Adequate hydration is essential for liver function and overall health.

★ Seniors should aim to drink plenty of water throughout the day and limit their intake of sugary beverages and caffeinated drinks.

★ Encourage portion control to prevent overeating and maintain a healthy weight.

★ Seniors should be mindful of portion sizes and listen to their body's hunger and fullness cues.

Balanced Macronutrients:

★ Emphasise the importance of balanced meals that include a combination of carbohydrates, proteins, and fats.

★ Seniors should aim for a balanced macronutrient distribution to support energy levels, stabilise blood sugar, and promote satiety.

Supplementation:

★ In some cases, seniors may benefit from dietary supplements to ensure they're meeting their nutritional needs, especially if they have specific deficiencies or dietary restrictions.

★ Consultation with a healthcare professional or registered dietitian can help determine appropriate supplementation based on individual health needs.

By following these nutritional guidelines, seniors can optimise their dietary habits to support liver health, manage fatty liver disease, and enhance overall quality of life.

Incorporating Essential Nutrients

Seniors diagnosed with fatty liver disease can benefit from incorporating essential nutrients into their diet to support liver health and manage the condition effectively. Here are key nutrients seniors should focus on:

1. ***Omega-3 Fatty Acids:*** Omega-3 fatty acids, found in fatty fish like salmon, mackerel, and sardines, as well as flaxseeds, chia seeds, and walnuts, have anti-inflammatory properties that can help reduce liver inflammation associated with fatty liver disease. Seniors should aim to include omega-3-rich foods in their diet regularly.

2. ***Vitamin E:*** Vitamin E is a powerful antioxidant that helps protect liver cells from damage caused by oxidative stress. Foods rich in vitamin E include almonds, sunflower seeds, spinach, broccoli, and avocado. Seniors can incorporate these foods into their meals and snacks to boost their vitamin E intake.

3. ***Vitamin C:*** Vitamin C is another antioxidant that supports liver health by neutralising harmful free radicals and reducing inflammation. Citrus fruits like

oranges, lemons, and grapefruits, as well as strawberries, bell peppers, and kiwi, are excellent sources of vitamin C that seniors can include in their diet.

4. **_Selenium:_** Selenium is a trace mineral with antioxidant properties that can help protect the liver from damage and support its detoxification processes. Seniors can obtain selenium from foods like Brazil nuts, seafood, poultry, eggs, and whole grains.

5. **_Zinc:_** Zinc plays a crucial role in liver function and helps support immune system function. Foods rich in zinc include lean meats, shellfish, legumes, nuts, seeds, and whole grains. Seniors should ensure they include zinc-rich foods in their diet regularly.

6. **_B-Vitamins:_** B-vitamins, including folate, B6, and B12, are important for liver health and metabolism. Seniors can obtain B-vitamins from a variety of foods, including leafy greens, fortified cereals, lean meats, poultry, fish, eggs, and dairy products.

7. **_Antioxidant-Rich Foods:_** Incorporating antioxidant-rich foods like berries, cherries, grapes, tomatoes, and dark leafy greens into the diet can help protect liver cells from oxidative damage and reduce inflammation associated with fatty liver disease.

8. ***Choline:*** Choline is a nutrient that plays a role in fat metabolism and liver function. Seniors can get choline from foods like eggs, lean meats, fish, cruciferous vegetables, and peanuts.

9. ***Fibre:*** Fibre aids in digestion and helps regulate blood sugar and cholesterol levels, which are important for managing fatty liver disease. Seniors should include plenty of fibre-rich foods like fruits, vegetables, whole grains, legumes, and nuts in their diet.

By incorporating these essential nutrients into their diet, seniors with fatty liver disease can support liver health, reduce inflammation, and improve overall well-being. It's important for seniors to focus on consuming a varied and nutrient-rich diet while limiting processed foods, sugar, and alcohol to effectively manage fatty liver disease. Consulting with a healthcare provider or registered dietitian can provide personalised guidance and recommendations based on individual health needs and preferences.

Meal Planning Strategies for Optimal Liver Health

Meal planning is a crucial aspect of managing liver health, especially for seniors with conditions like fatty liver disease. Here are some strategies to consider for creating balanced and liver-friendly meals:

Emphasise Whole Foods: Base meals around whole, unprocessed foods such as fruits, vegetables, whole grains, lean proteins, and healthy fats. These foods are rich in essential nutrients and antioxidants that support liver function and overall health.

Incorporate Lean Proteins: Include lean protein sources in each meal, such as poultry, fish, tofu, legumes, and low-fat dairy products. Protein is essential for tissue repair and helps maintain muscle mass, which is important for overall health and metabolism.

Opt for Healthy Fats: Choose healthy fats like those found in avocados, nuts, seeds, olive oil, and fatty fish. These fats contain omega-3 fatty acids, which have anti-inflammatory properties and support liver health. Limit the amount of saturated and trans fats in fried foods and processed snacks.

Balance Carbohydrates: Choose complex carbohydrates over refined carbohydrates. Whole grains like brown rice, quinoa, oats, and whole wheat bread provide fibre and nutrients while helping to regulate blood sugar levels. Limit intake of refined grains and sugars, which can contribute to insulin resistance and liver fat accumulation.

Include Fiber-Rich Foods: Incorporate plenty of fibre-rich foods into meals and snacks. Fibre helps promote satiety, regulate digestion, and support healthy cholesterol levels. Fruits, vegetables, legumes, and whole grains are excellent sources of dietary fibre.

Watch Portion Sizes: Be mindful of portion sizes to avoid overeating and excessive calorie intake. Use smaller plates and bowls to help reduce portion sizes, and pay attention to hunger and fullness signals.

Stay Hydrated: Drink plenty of water throughout the day to stay hydrated and support liver function. Water helps flush toxins from the body and aids in digestion and metabolism.

Limit Added Sugars and Processed Foods: Minimise consumption of foods and beverages high in added sugars, artificial sweeteners, and processed ingredients. These can increase liver fat buildup and inflammation.

Include Liver-Supportive Nutrients: Incorporate foods rich in liver-supportive nutrients such as vitamin E, vitamin C, selenium, zinc, and choline. These nutrients help protect liver cells from damage and support detoxification processes.

Plan Ahead and Prepare Meals: Take time to plan meals and snacks in advance to ensure they are balanced and nutritious. Batch cooking and meal prep can help save time and make it easier to stick to a healthy eating plan throughout the week.

Seek Professional Guidance: Consult with a healthcare provider or registered dietitian for personalised meal planning advice tailored to individual health needs and dietary preferences. They can provide guidance on nutrient requirements, portion control, and dietary adjustments to support optimal liver health.

By following these meal planning strategies, seniors can take proactive steps to support liver health, manage conditions like fatty liver disease, and promote overall well-being through nutrition and healthy eating habits.

CHAPTER FOUR

Building a Healthy Plate: Senior-Friendly Recipes

Creating nutritious and delicious meals is key to supporting liver health and overall well-being for seniors with fatty liver disease. In this chapter, we'll explore a variety of senior-friendly recipes designed to nourish the body and delight the taste buds:

Vegetable Stir-Fry:

→ Stir-fried vegetables with lean protein sources like tofu or chicken breast make for a satisfying and nutrient-dense meal.

→ Seniors can customise their stir-fry with their favourite vegetables and seasonings for a flavorful dish.

Quinoa Salad with Avocado and Chickpeas:

→ Quinoa is a versatile whole grain that serves as a nutritious base for salads.

→ Combine cooked quinoa with diced avocado, chickpeas, cherry tomatoes, and a squeeze of lemon juice for a refreshing and filling salad option.

→ Salmon is rich in omega-3 fatty acids, which have anti-inflammatory properties beneficial for liver health.

→ Bake seasoned salmon fillets alongside a medley of roasted vegetables, such as carrots, broccoli, and Brussels sprouts, for a simple yet satisfying meal.

Spinach and Mushroom Omelette:

→ Whisk together eggs with fresh spinach and sliced mushrooms for a nutritious and protein-packed omelette.

→ Seniors can customise their omelette with additional vegetables and herbs for added flavour and variety.

Mango and Black Bean Salsa:

→ Combine diced mango, black beans, red onion, cilantro, and lime juice for a vibrant and refreshing salsa.

→ Serve with whole grain tortilla chips or as a topping for grilled fish or chicken for a nutritious and flavorful meal option.

These senior-friendly recipes are not only delicious but also nutrient-dense, providing essential vitamins, minerals, and antioxidants to support liver health and overall vitality. Experimenting with new flavours and ingredients can make mealtime enjoyable and nourishing for seniors managing fatty liver disease.

Delicious and Nutritious Meal Ideas

Maintaining optimal liver health doesn't mean sacrificing flavour or variety in meals. Here are some delicious and nutritious meal ideas tailored to support liver health:

Breakfast:

1. **Avocado Toast with Poached Eggs:** Top whole-grain toast with mashed avocado, poached eggs, and a sprinkle of chia seeds. Avocado provides healthy fats, while eggs offer protein and essential nutrients.

2. **Greek Yoghurt Parfait:** Layer Greek yoghurt with mixed berries, almonds, and a drizzle of honey or maple syrup. Greek yoghurt is rich in protein and probiotics, while berries and nuts provide antioxidants and healthy fats.

Lunch:

3. **Quinoa Salad with Grilled Chicken:** Combine cooked quinoa with mixed greens, grilled chicken breast, cherry tomatoes, cucumber slices, and

avocado. Drizzle with olive oil and balsamic vinegar for a Flavourful dressing.

4. **Salmon and Avocado Wrap:** Fill a whole-grain wrap with grilled salmon, sliced avocado, spinach leaves, and a dollop of Greek yoghurt or tzatziki sauce. Serve with a side of carrot sticks or cucumber slices.

Dinner:

5. **Grilled Vegetable Stir-Fry:** Stir-fry a colourful mix of bell peppers, broccoli, snap peas, carrots, and mushrooms in olive oil and garlic. Add tofu or lean protein of choice and toss with a light soy sauce or teriyaki glaze. Serve over brown rice or quinoa.

6. **Baked Cod with Roasted Vegetables:** Season cod fillets with lemon juice, garlic, and herbs, then bake until flaky. Roast a medley of vegetables such as zucchini, bell peppers, onions, and cherry tomatoes tossed in olive oil and Italian seasoning.

Snacks:

7. **Almond Butter and Banana Slices:** Spread almond butter on whole-grain crackers or rice cakes and top with banana slices for a satisfying and nutritious snack rich in healthy fats and potassium.

8. **Vegetable Sticks with Hummus:** Dip crunchy vegetable sticks like carrots, cucumbers, and bell peppers into creamy hummus for a satisfying snack packed with fibre and protein.

Desserts:

9. **Baked Apples with Cinnamon:** Core apples and sprinkle with cinnamon and a touch of honey. Bake until tender and serve warm with a dollop of Greek yoghurt or a sprinkle of chopped nuts for a comforting dessert.

10. **Chia Seed Pudding:** Mix chia seeds with almond milk, vanilla extract, and a touch of maple syrup. Let it sit in the fridge until thickened, then top with fresh berries or sliced almonds for a nutritious and satisfying dessert option.

Beverages:

11. **Green Smoothie:** Blend spinach, kale, banana, pineapple, and a splash of coconut water for a refreshing and nutrient-packed green smoothie that supports liver health.

12. **Herbal Tea:** Enjoy a cup of herbal tea such as dandelion root, milk thistle, or ginger tea, which are known for their liver-cleansing properties and soothing effects.

These meal ideas are not only delicious but also nutrient-dense, providing essential vitamins, minerals, antioxidants, and healthy fats that support liver health and overall well-being. Incorporating a variety of colourful fruits, vegetables, whole grains, lean proteins, and healthy fats into meals and snacks can help seniors maintain optimal liver function and promote a healthy lifestyle.

Recipe Modifications for Liver-Friendly Eating

Modifying recipes to be liver-friendly involves making simple adjustments to reduce saturated fats, processed ingredients, and excessive sugars while increasing the intake of nutrient-dense foods that support liver health. Here are some recipe modifications to consider:

Reduce Saturated Fats:

- ➤ Replace saturated fats like butter and lard with healthier alternatives such as olive oil, avocado oil, or coconut oil.

- ➤ Trim visible fat from meats before cooking and opt for lean cuts of poultry, beef, or pork.

Incorporate Healthy Fats:

- ➤ Add sources of healthy fats like avocados, nuts, seeds, and fatty fish (salmon, mackerel) to recipes.

➢ Use nut butters or mashed avocado as spreads instead of butter or margarine.

Increase Fibre Content:

➢ Use whole grains like brown rice, quinoa, whole wheat pasta, or oats instead of refined grains.

➢ Add extra vegetables to recipes, such as spinach, kale, peppers, and carrots, to boost fibre content and nutrient density.

Limit Added Sugars:

➢ Substitute refined sugars with natural sweeteners like honey, maple syrup, or dates.

➢ Use ripe fruits like bananas, applesauce, or pureed dates to naturally sweeten baked goods and desserts.

Choose Lean Proteins:

➢ Opt for lean protein sources like skinless poultry, fish, tofu, tempeh, or legumes in place of fatty cuts of meat.

➢ Incorporate plant-based protein sources like beans, lentils, and chickpeas into soups, salads, and main dishes.

➢ Flavour dishes with herbs, spices, citrus juices, and vinegar instead of salt.

➢ Use low-sodium broth or homemade broth in soups and stews.

Use Cooking Methods Wisely:

➢ Use healthier cooking methods such as baking, grilling, steaming, or sautéing with little oil.

➢ Avoid deep-frying foods and opt for air frying or baking instead.

Boost Antioxidant Content:

➢ Include antioxidant-rich ingredients like berries, tomatoes, leafy greens, and colourful vegetables in salads, smoothies, and side dishes.

➢ Incorporate fresh herbs like parsley, cilantro, basil, and mint to add flavour and nutrients to recipes.

Emphasise Hydration:

➢ Encourage hydration by incorporating hydrating foods like cucumbers, watermelon, oranges, and celery into recipes.

➢ Offer infused water or herbal teas as refreshing beverage options.

Mindful Portion Control:

➢ Serve appropriately sized portions to prevent overeating and promote weight management.

➢ Use smaller plates and utensils to help control portion sizes and encourage mindful eating habits.

By implementing these recipe modifications, individuals can enjoy delicious and satisfying meals while supporting liver health and overall well-being. Experimenting with new ingredients, flavours, and cooking techniques can make the transition to liver-friendly eating both enjoyable and sustainable.

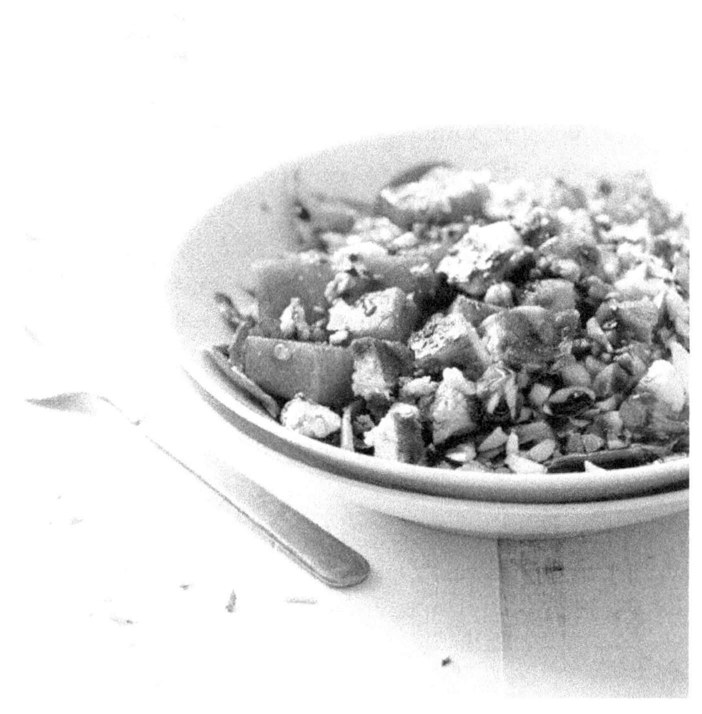

CHAPTER FIVE

Incorporating Superfoods into Your Diet Plan

Superfoods are nutrient-rich foods that offer a myriad of health benefits, including supporting liver health and combating inflammation. In this chapter, we'll explore a variety of superfoods that seniors can incorporate into their diet plan to promote liver health and overall well-being:

Turmeric:
- Turmeric includes curcumin, which has powerful anti-inflammatory and antioxidant properties.

- Seniors can add turmeric to soups, stews, curries, and smoothies for a vibrant colour and added health benefits.

Leafy Greens:
- Leafy greens such as spinach, kale, and Swiss chard are rich in vitamins, minerals, and phytonutrients that support liver detoxification and promote overall health.

- Seniors can enjoy leafy greens in salads, smoothies, stir-fries, and soups for a nutrient boost.

Berries:
- Berries like blueberries, strawberries, and raspberries are packed with antioxidants that help reduce inflammation and protect against oxidative stress.

- Seniors can enjoy berries as a topping for yoghurt, oatmeal, or cereal, or as a standalone snack.

Walnuts:
- Walnuts are a good source of omega-3 fatty acids, which have anti-inflammatory properties and support heart and brain health.

- Seniors can add walnuts to salads, oatmeal, baked goods, or enjoy them as a nutritious snack on their own.

Green Tea:
- Green tea contains catechins, powerful antioxidants known for their anti-inflammatory and liver-protective properties.

- Drinking green tea regularly may help reduce liver fat accumulation, improve liver function, and lower the risk of liver disease progression.

- Seniors can enjoy green tea as a refreshing beverage throughout the day or incorporate it into recipes such as smoothies and iced teas for added health benefits.

Cruciferous Vegetables:
- Cruciferous vegetables like broccoli, cauliflower, Brussels sprouts, and cabbage are rich in compounds that support liver detoxification and promote optimal liver function.

- These vegetables contain glucosinolates, which are sulphur-containing compounds that aid in the removal of toxins from the body and support the production of enzymes involved in detoxification processes.

- Seniors can include cruciferous vegetables in their meals by steaming, roasting, or stir-frying them as side dishes or incorporating them into salads and soups for added nutritional value.

Olive Oil:
- Olive oil is a heart-healthy fat rich in monounsaturated fatty acids and antioxidants, such as oleic acid and

polyphenols, which have been shown to reduce inflammation and improve liver health.

- Seniors can use olive oil as a primary cooking oil or drizzle it over salads, vegetables, and cooked dishes for added flavour and health benefits.

- Opt for extra virgin olive oil, which undergoes minimal processing and retains the highest levels of antioxidants and beneficial compounds.

Incorporating these superfoods into a balanced diet can provide seniors with essential nutrients, antioxidants, and bioactive compounds that support liver health, reduce inflammation, and promote overall well-being. By embracing the power of superfoods, seniors can take proactive steps towards managing fatty liver disease and optimising their health for the long term.

Exploring Nutrient-Rich Superfoods for Optimal Liver Health

Incorporating superfoods into your diet plan can significantly enhance liver health by providing essential nutrients, antioxidants, and anti-inflammatory compounds. Here are some nutrient-rich superfoods to consider adding to your diet:

1. **Leafy Greens:**

☐ Spinach, Kale, and Swiss Chard: Rich in chlorophyll, vitamins (A, C, K), minerals (iron, calcium), and antioxidants, leafy greens support liver detoxification processes and help reduce inflammation.

2. **Cruciferous Vegetables:**

☐ Broccoli, Brussels Sprouts, and Cauliflower: These vegetables contain compounds like sulforaphane and glucosinolates, which support liver detoxification and promote optimal liver function.

3. **Berries:**

☐ Blueberries, Strawberries, and Raspberries: Packed with antioxidants like anthocyanins, berries help protect liver cells from oxidative stress and inflammation, while also supporting overall health.

4. **Fatty Fish:**

☐ Salmon, Mackerel, and Sardines: High in omega-3 fatty acids, fatty fish help reduce inflammation, lower triglyceride levels, and improve liver fat metabolism.

5. <u>**Nuts and Seeds:**</u>

- ☐ Walnuts, Flaxseeds, and Chia Seeds: Rich in omega-3 fatty acids, fibre, and antioxidants, nuts and seeds support heart health and reduce inflammation in the liver.

6. <u>**Turmeric:**</u>

- ☐ This golden spice contains curcumin, a potent anti-inflammatory compound that helps protect liver cells from damage, reduce inflammation, and support liver detoxification pathways.

7. <u>**Garlic:**</u>

- ☐ Garlic contains sulphur compounds like allicin, which support liver detoxification and help reduce oxidative stress and inflammation in the liver.

8. <u>**Green Tea:**</u>

- ☐ Rich in catechins and antioxidants, green tea helps protect liver cells from damage, improve liver function, and reduce the risk of liver diseases like fatty liver disease.

9. <u>Avocado:</u>

- [ ] Avocado is a source of healthy fats, fibre, and antioxidants like vitamin E and glutathione, which support liver health, reduce inflammation, and promote detoxification.

10. <u>Beets:</u>

- [ ] Beets contain betalains, which support liver detoxification and help reduce inflammation. They are also rich in fibre, antioxidants, and folate, which promote overall health.

11. <u>Quinoa:</u>

- [ ] Quinoa is a nutrient-dense whole grain that provides protein, fibre, vitamins, and minerals. It supports stable blood sugar levels and helps maintain a healthy weight, which is important for liver health.

12. <u>Greek Yoghurt:</u>

- [ ] Greek Yoghurt is rich in probiotics, protein, and calcium. It supports gut health, which is linked to liver health, and provides essential nutrients for overall well-being.

Incorporating these nutrient-rich superfoods into your diet can help support liver health, reduce inflammation, and protect against liver diseases. Try incorporating a variety of these superfoods into your meals and snacks to maximise their health benefits and promote optimal liver function. Remember to balance your diet with a variety of nutrient-dense foods and consult with a healthcare provider or registered dietitian for personalised dietary recommendations based on your individual health needs and goals.

Recipes Featuring Liver-Supportive Ingredients

Incorporating liver-supportive ingredients into your recipes can promote optimal liver health and overall well-being. Here are some delicious and nutritious recipes featuring nutrient-rich foods known for their liver-supportive properties:

1. Superfood Spinach Salad:

Ingredients:

- Fresh spinach leaves
- Sliced strawberries
- Blueberries
- Sliced almonds
- Crumbled feta cheese (optional)
- Dressing:
- Olive oil

* Balsamic vinegar
* Dijon mustard
* Honey (optional)

Instructions:

1. In a large bowl, combine spinach, strawberries, blueberries, almonds, and feta cheese.

2. In a small jar, mix olive oil, balsamic vinegar, Dijon mustard, and honey to taste to create the dressing.

3. Drizzle the salad with the dressing and gently toss to coat. Serve immediately.

2. Turmeric-Garlic Roasted Vegetables:

Ingredients:

* Mixed veggies (broccoli, cauliflower, carrots, and bell peppers)
* Olive oil
* Minced garlic
* Ground turmeric
* Salt and pepper to taste

Instructions:

1. Preheat the oven to 400 degrees Fahrenheit (200 degrees Celsius) and line a baking sheet with parchment paper.

2. Chop the vegetables into bite-sized pieces and place them on the prepared baking sheet.

3. In a small bowl, mix olive oil, minced garlic, ground turmeric, salt, and pepper.

4. Drizzle the oil mixture over the vegetables and toss to coat evenly.

5. Roast in the preheated oven for 20-25 minutes or until the vegetables are tender and golden brown.

3. Baked Salmon with Lemon and Dill:

Ingredients:

- ❖ Salmon fillets
- ❖ Lemon slices
- ❖ Fresh dill
- ❖ Olive oil
- ❖ Garlic powder
- ❖ Salt and pepper to taste

Instructions:

1. Preheat the oven to 375°F (190°C) and line a baking dish with parchment paper.

2. Place the salmon fillets in the baking dish and season with garlic powder, salt, and pepper.

3. Drizzle olive oil over the salmon and top with lemon slices and fresh dill.

4. Bake in the preheated oven for 15-20 minutes or until the salmon is cooked through and flakes easily with a fork.

Ingredients:

- Spinach leaves
- Frozen mixed berries
- Plain Greek yoghourt
- Green tea (brewed and cooled)
- Honey or maple syrup (optional)

Instructions:

1. In a blender, combine spinach leaves, frozen mixed berries, Greek yoghurt, and cooled green tea.

2. Blend until smooth and creamy, adding honey or maple syrup for sweetness if desired.

3. Pour into glasses and serve immediately as a refreshing and liver-supportive smoothie.

5. Quinoa and Beet Salad:

Ingredients:

- ☐ Cooked quinoa
- ☐ Roasted beets (sliced)
- ☐ Baby spinach leaves
- ☐ Crumbled goat cheese
- ☐ Chopped walnuts
- ☐ Balsamic vinaigrette dressing

Instructions:

1. In a large bowl, combine cooked quinoa, roasted beets, baby spinach leaves, crumbled goat cheese, and chopped walnuts.
2. Drizzle with balsamic vinaigrette dressing and toss gently to combine.
3. Serve as a hearty and nutritious salad packed with liver-supportive ingredients.

Incorporating these recipes into your meal plan can help support liver health and provide a delicious way to enjoy nutrient-rich foods that promote overall well-being. Experiment with different combinations of liver-supportive ingredients to create flavorful and satisfying dishes that nourish your body and support optimal liver function.

CHAPTER SIX

Meal Planning and Preparation Tips for Seniors

Meal planning and preparation can significantly impact the dietary habits and overall health of seniors managing fatty liver disease. In this chapter, we'll explore practical meal planning and preparation tips tailored specifically for seniors:

Plan Balanced Meals:

- ★ Seniors should aim to include a variety of nutrient-dense foods in their meals, including fruits, vegetables, whole grains, lean proteins, and healthy fats.

- ★ Planning meals ahead of time can help ensure balanced nutrition and prevent reliance on convenience foods high in unhealthy fats and sugars.

Batch Cooking and Freezing:

- ★ Seniors can save time and effort by preparing large batches of meals and portioning them into individual servings for later use.

★ Freezing meals in portion-sized containers allows for easy reheating and minimises food waste.

★ Kitchen appliances such as slow cookers, pressure cookers, and air fryers can streamline meal preparation and make cooking more accessible for seniors.

★ These appliances require minimal hands-on time and can help tenderise tough cuts of meat and enhance flavours.

★ Encourage seniors to explore new recipes and flavours to keep mealtime exciting and enjoyable.

★ Trying new ingredients and cooking techniques can broaden culinary horizons and make healthy eating more sustainable in the long term.

★ Take into account individual dietary preferences, allergies, and restrictions when planning meals for seniors.

★ Flexibility and customization ensure that meals are both nutritious and enjoyable for seniors managing fatty liver disease.

By incorporating these meal planning and preparation tips into their routine, seniors can simplify the cooking process, maintain a healthy diet, and support liver health for optimal well-being.

Practical Strategies for Meal Planning

Meal planning is a key component of maintaining a nutritious diet that supports liver health. Here are some practical strategies to help you plan and prepare liver-friendly meals:

1. Set Aside Time for Planning:
   - Dedicate a specific time each week to plan your meals. This could be on a weekend or whichever day works best for you.

2. Consider Your Schedule:
   - Take into account your schedule for the upcoming week, including work commitments, appointments, and any social activities that may impact meal times.

3. Start with a Template:
   - Use a meal planning template or calendar to map out your meals for the week. Include breakfast, lunch, dinner, and snacks.

4. Focus on Balanced Meals:

- Aim to include a variety of nutrient-rich foods in each meal, including lean proteins, whole grains, healthy fats, and plenty of fruits and vegetables.

5. Plan for Leftovers:

- Make larger batches of recipes so you can enjoy leftovers for lunch or dinner later in the week. This can save time and reduce food waste.

6. Take Inventory:

- Before heading to the grocery store, take inventory of ingredients you already have on hand. This will help you avoid buying unnecessary items and ensure you have everything you need for your planned meals.

7. Create a Shopping List:

- Based on your meal plan and inventory, create a shopping list of the items you need to purchase. Organise the list by categories (e.g., produce, dairy, pantry staples) to make shopping more efficient.

8. Choose Convenient Options:

- Opt for convenience foods like pre-cut vegetables, frozen fruits, and pre-cooked grains to save time during meal preparation.

9. Include Liver-Supportive Foods:

- Incorporate liver-supportive ingredients such as leafy greens, cruciferous vegetables, fatty fish, nuts, seeds, and whole grains into your meals and snacks.

10. Batch Cooking:
   - Spend a few hours on your designated meal prep day to cook and prepare ingredients in advance. This can include washing and chopping vegetables, cooking grains and proteins, and assembling meals for the week.

11. Stay Flexible:
   - Be open to making adjustments to your meal plan based on changes in your schedule or preferences. Flexibility is key to sticking to your plan and enjoying the process of meal planning.

12. Experiment with New Recipes:
   - Try incorporating new recipes and flavours into your meal plan to keep things interesting and enjoyable. To broaden your culinary horizons, experiment with new dishes and cooking methods.

13. Listen to Your Body:
   - Pay attention to hunger and fullness cues, as well as any dietary preferences or restrictions you may have. Adjust your meal plan accordingly to ensure it meets your nutritional needs and tastes.

By implementing these practical strategies for meal planning, you can streamline the process of preparing liver-friendly meals while promoting overall health and well-being. Consistency and organisation are key to successfully incorporating nutritious foods into your diet and supporting optimal liver function over time.

Time-Saving Meal Preparation Techniques

Meal preparation can be made more efficient and convenient, especially for seniors managing a fatty liver diet. Here are some time-saving techniques to streamline the cooking process:

1. ***Batch Cooking:***
   - Dedicate a day or two each week to batch-cook staple ingredients like grains (quinoa, brown rice), proteins (chicken breast, tofu), and vegetables (roasted sweet potatoes, steamed broccoli). Store them in portioned containers for quick and easy meal assembly throughout the week.

2. ***One-Pot Meals:***
   - Prepare meals that can be cooked in a single pot or pan, minimising cleanup time. Recipes like soups, stews, stir-fries, and skillet meals are excellent options for efficient cooking and easy cleanup.

3. ***Slow Cooker or Instant Pot Meals:***
   - Utilise slow cookers or Instant Pots to prepare hands-off meals with minimal effort. Simply add ingredients to the appliance in the morning and return to a delicious meal by dinnertime.

4. ***Pre-cut and Pre-packaged Ingredients:***
   - Purchase pre-cut vegetables, pre-washed greens, and pre-packaged salads to reduce prep time. These convenient options can save valuable time in the kitchen without sacrificing nutrition.

5. ***Frozen Fruits and Vegetables:***
   - Stock up on frozen fruits and vegetables, which are pre-cut and require no preparation. They can be easily incorporated into smoothies, stir-fries, and soups for a quick and nutritious addition to meals.

6. ***Meal Kits or Pre-prepared Meals:***
   - Consider subscribing to meal kit services or purchasing pre-prepared meals designed for seniors. These options provide pre-portioned ingredients and recipes, saving time on meal planning, shopping, and cooking.

7. ***Multi-tasking Cooking:***
   - Maximise efficiency by multi-tasking during meal preparation. For example, while a pot of quinoa is cooking, you can chop vegetables or prepare a salad to accompany the meal.

8. ***Utilise Convenience Appliances:***
   - Invest in time-saving kitchen appliances like food processors, vegetable spiralizers, and rice cookers to expedite meal preparation and simplify cooking tasks.

9. *Prep Ingredients in Advance:*
   - Wash, peel, and chop vegetables in advance and store them in airtight containers in the refrigerator. This allows for quicker meal assembly during busy weekdays.

10. *Plan Simple Meals:*
   - Opt for simple recipes with minimal ingredients and preparation steps. Focus on nutrient-dense meals that can be prepared quickly without compromising flavour or nutrition.

11. *Leftovers for Future Meals:*
   - Cook larger portions than needed and save leftovers for future meals. Leftovers can be refrigerated or frozen for later use, providing convenient options for busy days or evenings.

12. *Cook Once, Eat Twice:*
   - Transform leftovers into fresh meals to reduce food waste and save time. For example, roasted vegetables can be added to salads, wraps, or omelettes for a quick and nutritious meal.

By incorporating these time-saving meal preparation techniques into your routine, seniors can enjoy delicious and nutritious meals without spending excessive time in the kitchen. Planning ahead, utilising convenience options, and simplifying cooking processes can make mealtime more enjoyable and stress-free while supporting a fatty liver diet.

CHAPTER SEVEN

Lifestyle Changes for Managing Fatty Liver

In addition to dietary modifications, certain lifestyle changes can play a significant role in managing fatty liver disease and promoting liver health. In this chapter, we'll explore key lifestyle changes that seniors can implement to support their liver health:

Regular Physical Activity:

  - Engaging in regular physical activity can help seniors manage weight, improve insulin sensitivity, and reduce liver fat accumulation.

  - Encourage seniors to incorporate activities they enjoy, such as walking, swimming, yoga, or tai chi, into their daily routine.

Maintain a Healthy Weight:

  - Achieving and maintaining a healthy weight is essential for liver health and overall well-being.

  - Seniors should focus on gradual weight loss through a combination of dietary changes, physical activity, and lifestyle modifications.

- Chronic stress can contribute to inflammation and exacerbate fatty liver disease.

- Encourage seniors to practise stress-reducing techniques such as meditation, deep breathing exercises, mindfulness, and spending time in nature.

Quality Sleep:

- Adequate sleep is crucial for liver health and overall vitality.

- Seniors should aim for seven to eight hours of quality sleep per night and establish a regular sleep schedule to optimise their restorative sleep patterns.

Limit Exposure to Toxins:

- Seniors should be mindful of environmental toxins and pollutants that can impact liver health.

- Minimise exposure to harmful substances such as cigarette smoke, alcohol, pesticides, and industrial chemicals to reduce liver burden.

By adopting these lifestyle changes, seniors can enhance their overall health and well-being while effectively managing fatty liver disease for long-term liver health.

Importance of Physical Activity and Stress Management for Seniors with Fatty Liver

Physical activity and stress management are crucial components of a comprehensive approach to managing fatty liver disease in seniors. Here's why they are important:

Physical Activity:

1. **Weight Management:** Regular physical activity helps maintain a healthy weight or achieve weight loss, which is essential for managing fatty liver disease. Losing excess weight can reduce liver fat accumulation and improve liver function.

2. **Improved Insulin Sensitivity:** Exercise helps improve insulin sensitivity, reducing the risk of insulin resistance and diabetes, both of which are common risk factors for fatty liver disease.

3. **Enhanced Liver Health:** Physical activity promotes blood circulation and oxygen delivery to liver cells, supporting liver function and promoting detoxification processes.

4. **Reduced Inflammation:** Exercise has anti-inflammatory effects on the body, which can help reduce liver inflammation and prevent disease progression.

5. **Increased Energy Levels:** Regular physical activity can boost energy levels, improve mood, and enhance overall quality of life for seniors managing fatty liver disease.

Stress Management:

1. **Reduced Cortisol Levels:** Chronic stress can elevate cortisol levels, which may contribute to inflammation and liver damage. Implementing stress management techniques can help lower cortisol levels and protect liver health.

2. **Improved Mental Well-being:** Stress management techniques such as meditation, deep breathing exercises, and mindfulness can help reduce anxiety, depression, and overall stress levels, promoting mental well-being in seniors.

3. **Healthy Coping Mechanisms:** Seniors can learn healthy coping mechanisms to deal with stressors and challenges in life, reducing the likelihood of turning to unhealthy behaviours like overeating or excessive alcohol consumption, which can worsen fatty liver disease.

4. **Better Sleep Quality:** Stress management practices can improve sleep quality and duration, which is essential for overall health and liver function.

5. **Enhanced Immune Function:** Chronic stress weakens the immune system, making individuals more susceptible to infections and illnesses. Managing stress can help strengthen the immune system and promote better health outcomes.

Combined Approach:

1. **Synergistic Benefits:** Combining regular physical activity with stress management techniques can have synergistic benefits for seniors managing fatty liver disease. Together, they can improve overall health, reduce inflammation, and promote liver function.

2. **Holistic Approach to Wellness:** Physical activity and stress management are integral components of a holistic approach to wellness for seniors. By addressing both physical and emotional aspects of health, seniors can better manage fatty liver disease and improve their overall quality of life.

Incorporating regular physical activity and stress management techniques into daily life can play a significant role in managing fatty liver disease and promoting overall health and well-being for seniors. It's important for seniors to work with healthcare providers and consider individual preferences and limitations when developing a personalised plan for physical activity and stress management.

Enhancing Quality of Life Through Lifestyle Modifications

Lifestyle modifications play a vital role in enhancing the quality of life for seniors managing fatty liver disease. By adopting healthy habits and making positive changes to their daily routines, seniors can improve liver health, manage symptoms, and promote overall well-being. Here's how lifestyle modifications can enhance quality of life:

<u>Healthy Eating Habits:</u>

   - Following a balanced diet rich in fruits, vegetables, whole grains, lean proteins, and healthy fats can support liver health and reduce the progression of fatty liver disease.

   - Limiting intake of processed foods, saturated fats, sugars, and alcohol can help manage symptoms and improve liver function.

<u>Regular Physical Activity:</u>

   - Engaging in regular exercise, such as walking, swimming, yoga, or tai chi, can improve circulation, reduce inflammation, and promote weight loss or weight management.

- Exercise also enhances mood, increases energy levels, and improves overall physical and mental well-being.

Maintaining a Healthy Weight:

- Achieving and maintaining a healthy weight through diet and exercise can reduce liver fat accumulation and improve liver function.

- Weight loss, if necessary, can significantly reduce the risk of complications associated with fatty liver disease.

Stress Management:

- Practising stress management techniques like meditation, deep breathing exercises, yoga, or mindfulness can help reduce cortisol levels, lower inflammation, and improve liver health.

- Managing stress effectively can also enhance mental well-being and improve overall quality of life.

Adequate Sleep:

- Prioritising good sleep hygiene and ensuring adequate rest can support liver health and overall well-being.

- Establishing a regular sleep schedule, creating a relaxing bedtime routine, and minimising screen time before bed can promote better sleep quality.

Hydration:

- Staying hydrated by drinking plenty of water throughout the day supports liver function and helps flush toxins from the body.

- Limiting consumption of sugary beverages and alcohol is important for liver health.

Regular Medical Check-ups:

- Seniors should schedule regular check-ups with their healthcare providers to monitor liver function, assess disease progression, and adjust treatment plans as needed.

- Routine screenings for conditions like diabetes, high blood pressure, and cholesterol levels are also important for managing fatty liver disease and overall health.

Social Support:

- Maintaining social connections and seeking support from family, friends, or support groups can reduce feelings of isolation and improve mental well-being.

- Engaging in social activities and hobbies can provide a sense of purpose and fulfilment, enhancing overall quality of life.

Continued Education and Advocacy:

- Seniors should stay informed about fatty liver disease, its symptoms, treatment options, and lifestyle recommendations.

- Advocating for their own health care needs and communicating openly with healthcare providers can ensure they receive the best possible care and support.

By implementing these lifestyle modifications, seniors with fatty liver disease can enhance their quality of life, manage symptoms effectively, and promote overall health and well-being. It's important for seniors to work closely with healthcare providers to develop personalised lifestyle plans tailored to their individual needs and preferences.

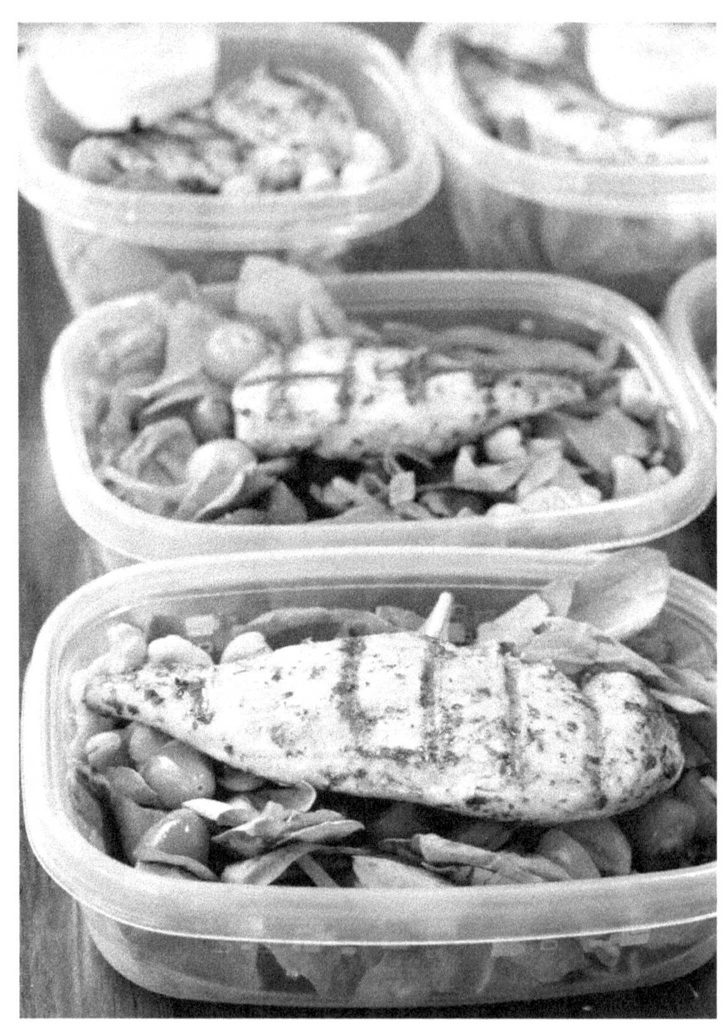

CHAPTER EIGHT

Exercise Regimen for Seniors with Fatty Liver

Regular exercise is an integral component of fatty liver management for seniors. In this chapter, we'll explore an exercise regimen specifically designed to support liver health and improve overall fitness for seniors:

Aerobic Exercise:

- Aerobic exercise, such as brisk walking, cycling, swimming, or dancing, helps improve cardiovascular health, burn calories, and reduce liver fat.

- Seniors should aim for at least 150 minutes of moderate-intensity aerobic exercise per week, spread out over several days.

Strength Training:

- Strength training exercises help build muscle mass, increase metabolism, and improve insulin sensitivity.

- Seniors can incorporate resistance bands, dumbbells, or bodyweight exercises into their routine to strengthen major muscle groups.

Flexibility and Balance Exercises:

- Flexibility and balance exercises, such as yoga, tai chi, or gentle stretching, help improve mobility, reduce the risk of falls, and promote overall well-being.

- Seniors should include flexibility and balance exercises in their weekly routine to maintain mobility and independence.

Progression and Adaptation:

- Seniors should start slowly and gradually increase the intensity and duration of their exercise regimen as tolerated.

- It's important to listen to the body's cues and adapt the exercise routine based on individual fitness levels and health conditions.

Be Hydrated and Listen to Your Body:

- Seniors should stay hydrated before, during, and after exercise to prevent dehydration and support optimal performance.

- It's essential to listen to the body's signals and adjust the intensity or duration of exercise as needed to avoid overexertion and injury.

By incorporating a balanced exercise regimen into their lifestyle, seniors can improve liver health, enhance physical fitness, and enjoy a higher quality of life.

Aerobic, Strength, and Flexibility Exercises

Incorporating a variety of exercises into a fitness routine can greatly benefit seniors managing fatty liver disease. Aerobic, strength, and flexibility exercises each offer unique advantages that contribute to overall health and well-being. Here's how they can be beneficial:

1. Aerobic Exercises:

Aerobic exercises, also known as cardio exercises, are activities that increase the heart rate and improve cardiovascular health. These exercises help burn calories, reduce body fat, and improve insulin sensitivity, all of which are important for managing fatty liver disease. Examples of aerobic exercises suitable for seniors include:

- Walking: A low-impact activity that can be easily incorporated into daily life. Seniors can walk outdoors or on a treadmill at a comfortable pace.

- Swimming: A relaxing, full-body workout that is low-impact on the joints. Swimming improves cardiovascular health and strengthens muscles.

- Cycling: Riding a stationary bike or going for a bike ride outdoors can improve heart health, increase stamina, and burn calories.

- Dancing: A fun and social way to get aerobic exercise. Dance classes tailored to seniors can improve balance, coordination, and cardiovascular health.

2. Strength Training:

Strength training workouts aim to increase muscle strength and endurance. Strength training is important for seniors to maintain muscle mass, bone density, and functional independence. It also helps boost metabolism and improve insulin sensitivity. Examples of strength training exercises for seniors include:

- Bodyweight Exercises: Squats, lunges, push-ups, and planks are effective bodyweight exercises that can be modified to suit different fitness levels.

- Resistance Band Exercises: Resistance bands offer gentle resistance and can be used to perform exercises that target various muscle groups.

- Weightlifting: Using light dumbbells or weight machines under supervision can help seniors build muscle strength and improve overall fitness.

3. Flexibility Exercises:

Flexibility exercises focus on improving joint mobility, range of motion, and overall flexibility. These exercises can help seniors maintain independence, prevent injuries, and reduce muscle tension and stiffness. Examples of flexibility exercises for seniors are:

- Yoga: Gentle yoga poses and stretches improve flexibility, balance, and relaxation. Yoga classes specifically designed for seniors can accommodate different fitness levels and abilities.

- Tai Chi: An ancient Chinese martial art that emphasises slow, flowing movements and deep breathing. Tai Chi promotes balance, flexibility, and mental attention.

- Stretching: Performing stretches for major muscle groups can improve flexibility and range of motion. Seniors should stretch slowly and gently, holding each stretch for 15-30 seconds.

Tips for Safe Exercise:

- Seniors should consult with their healthcare provider before starting any new exercise program, especially if they have underlying health conditions.

- Start slowly and gradually increase the intensity and duration of exercise sessions.

- Listen to your body and discontinue exercise if you feel pain, dizziness, or shortness of breath.

- Stay hydrated and dress appropriately for the weather and activity level.

- Warm up before exercise with gentle movements and cool down afterward with stretches to prevent injury.

Incorporating a combination of aerobic, strength, and flexibility exercises into a fitness routine can help seniors manage fatty liver disease, improve overall health, and enhance quality of life. By staying active and engaging in regular physical activity, seniors can enjoy better health outcomes and maintain independence as they age.

Creating a Personalised Exercise Routine for Liver Health

Designing a personalised exercise routine tailored to liver health involves considering individual fitness levels, preferences, and any existing medical conditions. Here's how seniors with fatty liver disease can create a safe and effective exercise plan:

Consult with Healthcare Providers:
   - Before starting any exercise program, seniors should consult with their healthcare providers, including their primary care physician and

specialists. They can provide valuable insights into specific health considerations and recommend appropriate exercise guidelines.

Assess Current Fitness Level:

- Seniors should assess their current fitness level, taking into account factors such as strength, flexibility, endurance, and balance. This assessment can help determine the appropriate starting point for their exercise routine.

Set Realistic Goals:

- Establish achievable goals based on individual health status, preferences, and lifestyle. Goals may include improving cardiovascular fitness, increasing muscle strength, enhancing flexibility, or simply maintaining overall health and well-being.

Incorporate Variety:

- Include a variety of aerobic, strength, and flexibility exercises to promote overall fitness and target different aspects of health. Variety also helps prevent boredom and reduces the risk of overuse injuries.

Choose Suitable Activities:

- Select exercises that are enjoyable, accessible, and appropriate for individual fitness levels. Low-impact activities such as walking, swimming, cycling, and gentle yoga are excellent choices for seniors with fatty liver disease.

Gradually Increase Intensity:

- Gradually increase the intensity, duration, and frequency of exercise sessions over time. Start with shorter sessions and lower intensity levels, then gradually progress as fitness improves and tolerance increases.

Include Strength Training:

- Incorporate strength training exercises at least two days per week to build muscle strength, improve bone density, and support overall health. To target main muscle groups, work with light weights, resistance bands, or bodyweight exercises.

Prioritise Flexibility and Balance:

- Allocate time for flexibility and balance exercises to improve joint mobility, reduce stiffness, and enhance stability. Include stretching, yoga, tai chi, or Pilates exercises to promote flexibility and balance.

Listen to Your Body:

- Pay attention to how your body reacts to exercise and modify your regimen accordingly. If you experience pain, discomfort, or excessive fatigue, modify your activities or seek guidance from a fitness professional.

Stay Consistent:

- Consistency is key to reaping the benefits of exercise for liver health. Aim for regular, consistent exercise sessions, even if they're shorter in duration. Incorporating physical activity into daily routines can help maintain momentum and foster long-term adherence.

Monitor Progress and Adjustments:

   - Keep track of progress by monitoring fitness improvements, changes in energy levels, and overall well-being. Adjust the exercise routine as needed to accommodate changes in health status, goals, or preferences.

Hydrate and Rest:

   - Stay hydrated before, during, and after exercise to maximise performance and recovery. Allow adequate time for rest and recovery between exercise sessions to prevent fatigue and minimise the risk of injury.

By creating a personalised exercise routine tailored to liver health, seniors with fatty liver disease can improve overall fitness, manage symptoms, and enhance quality of life. Consistent engagement in physical activity, combined with other healthy lifestyle habits, can support liver function and promote long-term well-being.

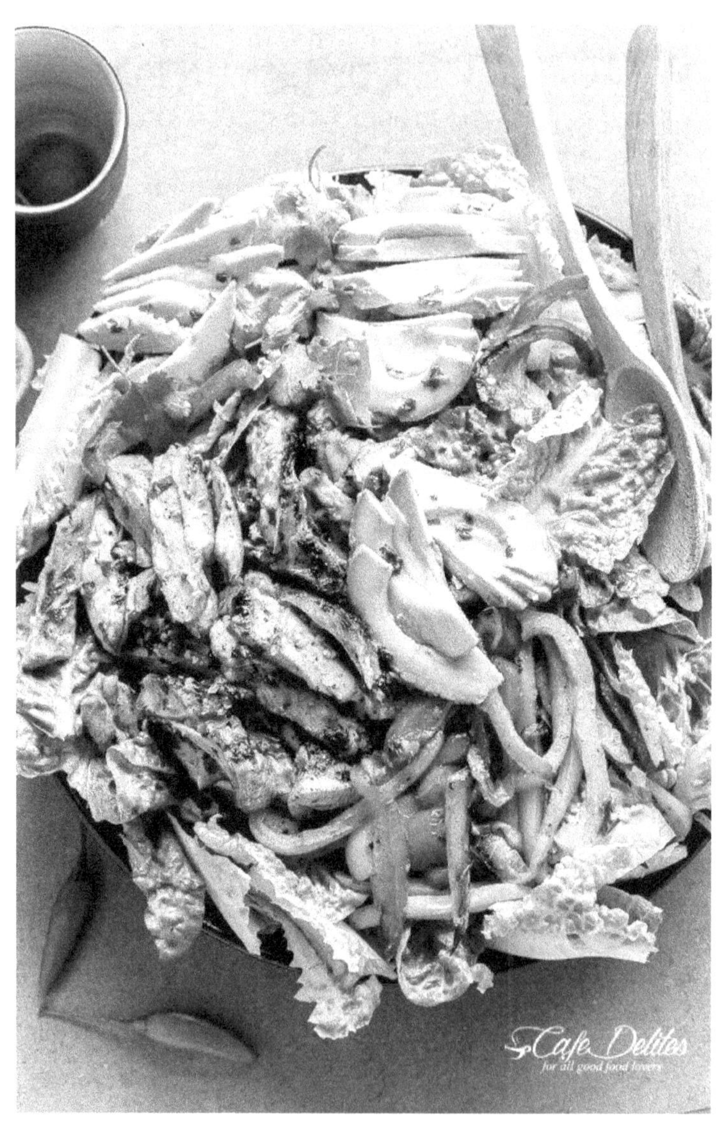
Cafe Delites
for all good food lovers

CHAPTER NINE

Managing Stress and Mental Health in Fatty Liver Management

Stress management and mental well-being are integral components of holistic fatty liver management for seniors. In this chapter, we'll explore strategies for effectively managing stress and supporting mental health:

1. Mindfulness and Meditation:
   - Practising mindfulness and meditation techniques can help seniors reduce stress, cultivate inner peace, and enhance emotional resilience.

   - Encourage seniors to dedicate a few minutes each day to mindfulness meditation, deep breathing exercises, or guided relaxation techniques.

2. Engage in Leisure Activities:
   - Engaging in enjoyable leisure activities, hobbies, and social interactions can help seniors alleviate stress, foster a sense of connection, and promote overall well-being.

   - Encourage seniors to pursue activities they love, whether it's gardening, painting, listening to music, or spending time with loved ones.

3. Seek Support:
   - Seniors should feel empowered to seek support from family members, friends, support groups, or mental health professionals when needed.

   - Sharing concerns, seeking guidance, and connecting with others who understand can provide valuable emotional support and coping resources.

4. Maintain a Positive Outlook:
   - Encourage seniors to cultivate a positive mindset and focus on gratitude, optimism, and resilience in the face of challenges.

   - Practising positive self-talk, reframing negative thoughts, and celebrating small victories can help seniors maintain a hopeful outlook and navigate fatty liver management with confidence.

5. Prioritise Self-Care:
   - Self-care practices, such as adequate sleep, regular physical activity, healthy nutrition, and relaxation techniques, are essential for maintaining mental and emotional well-being.

   - Seniors should prioritise self-care activities that nourish the mind, body, and spirit and make time for rest, relaxation, and rejuvenation.

By prioritising stress management and mental health, seniors can enhance their overall quality of life and better cope with the challenges of managing fatty liver disease.

Strategies for Stress Reduction and Emotional Well-Being

Managing stress and promoting emotional well-being are essential components of a holistic approach to managing fatty liver disease in seniors. Here are strategies to reduce stress and enhance emotional well-being:

1. Mindfulness Meditation:
   - Practise mindfulness meditation to cultivate awareness of the present moment, reduce stress, and promote relaxation. Seniors can participate in guided meditation sessions or use mindfulness apps for support

2. Deep Breathing Exercises:
   - Incorporate deep breathing exercises into daily routines to activate the body's relaxation response, reduce anxiety, and promote calmness. Seniors can practise deep breathing techniques throughout the day or during stressful situations.

3. Engage in Relaxation Techniques:
   - Explore relaxation techniques such as progressive muscle relaxation, visualisation, or guided imagery to alleviate tension, promote relaxation, and reduce stress levels.

4. Stay Active:

   - Engage in regular physical activity, such as walking, swimming, or yoga, to release endorphins, improve mood, and reduce symptoms of stress and anxiety.

5. Foster Social Connections:

   - Maintain social connections with family, friends, and community members to reduce feelings of loneliness and isolation. Seniors can participate in social activities, join clubs or groups, or volunteer in their communities.

6. Express Gratitude:

   - Practise gratitude by reflecting on and expressing appreciation for the positive aspects of life. Keeping a gratitude journal or sharing moments of gratitude with others can enhance emotional well-being and perspective.

7. Seek Support:

   - Reach out to loved ones, support groups, or mental health professionals for emotional support and guidance. Seniors can benefit from sharing their experiences, feelings, and concerns with trusted individuals who can offer empathy and understanding.

8. Limit Exposure to Stressors:

   - Identify sources of stress and take proactive steps to minimise exposure to stressors whenever possible. Seniors can set boundaries, prioritise tasks, and delegate responsibilities to reduce feelings of overwhelm and stress.

9. Practise Self-Care:
   - Prioritise self-care activities that improve physical, mental, and emotional health. Engage in activities that bring joy and relaxation, such as hobbies, reading, gardening, or spending time in nature.

10. Maintain a Healthy Lifestyle:
   - Follow a balanced diet, engage in regular physical activity, get adequate sleep, and avoid excessive alcohol consumption and smoking. A healthy lifestyle promotes overall well-being and resilience to stress.

11. Stay Informed and Proactive:
   - Stay informed about fatty liver disease, treatment options, and lifestyle recommendations. Take an active role in managing health by attending medical appointments, asking questions, and advocating for personal needs and preferences.

12. Practice Acceptance and Resilience:
   - Cultivate acceptance and resilience by acknowledging challenges, adapting to changes, and focusing on solutions rather than dwelling on setbacks. Seniors can develop coping skills to navigate life's ups and downs with grace and resilience.

By implementing these strategies for stress reduction and emotional well-being, seniors with fatty liver disease can enhance their overall quality of life, improve coping skills, and foster greater resilience in the face of challenges. It's important for seniors to prioritise self-care and seek support when needed to promote emotional wellness and long-term health.

Importance of Mental Health Support for Seniors with Fatty Liver

Mental health support is essential for seniors managing fatty liver disease as it addresses the emotional and psychological aspects of their well-being. Here's why mental health support is important:

Emotional Resilience:

   - Dealing with a chronic condition like fatty liver disease can be challenging and may lead to feelings of stress, anxiety, or depression. Mental health support equips seniors with coping mechanisms and resilience to navigate these emotional challenges effectively.

Quality of Life:

   - Addressing mental health concerns contributes to an improved quality of life for seniors. By managing stress, anxiety, and depression, seniors can enjoy a greater sense of well-being, fulfilment, and satisfaction in their daily lives.

Adherence to Treatment Plans:

   - Seniors who receive mental health support are more likely to adhere to their treatment plans and engage in healthy lifestyle behaviours. Improved adherence leads to better management of fatty liver disease and reduced risk of complications.

Social Support:

   - Mental health support provides seniors with opportunities to connect with others who may be experiencing similar challenges. Peer support groups, therapy sessions, or support networks offer a sense of belonging, validation, and understanding.

Coping Strategies:

   - Mental health support equips seniors with effective coping strategies to manage stress, cope with uncertainty, and navigate life's challenges. Seniors learn valuable skills to regulate emotions, problem-solve, and adapt to changes in health or circumstances.

Enhanced Communication:

   - Engaging in therapy or counselling sessions encourages open communication and expression of thoughts and feelings. Seniors learn to articulate their needs, concerns, and preferences, leading to improved relationships and support systems.

Reduced Isolation and Loneliness:

  - Fatty liver disease or related symptoms may limit seniors' ability to engage in social activities or maintain social connections. Mental health support provides a safe space for seniors to combat feelings of isolation, loneliness, and disconnection.

Early Intervention and Prevention:

  - Mental health support facilitates early intervention and prevention of more severe mental health issues. By addressing symptoms of stress, anxiety, or depression early on, seniors can prevent escalation and mitigate the impact on their overall health.

Improved Cognitive Function:

  - Managing mental health concerns can have positive effects on cognitive function and overall brain health in seniors. Emotional well-being is closely linked to cognitive function, memory, and decision-making abilities.

Holistic Approach to Health:

  - Fatty liver disease affects not only the physical body but also mental and emotional aspects of health. Mental health support complements medical treatment by addressing the holistic needs of seniors, promoting overall wellness and healing.

Empowerment and Self-Advocacy:

- Seniors who receive mental health support feel empowered to take an active role in their health care journey. They become advocates for their own well-being, make informed decisions, and assert their needs and preferences confidently.

Long-Term Well-Being:

- Prioritising mental health support sets the foundation for long-term well-being and resilience in seniors with fatty liver disease. It fosters a positive outlook, strengthens coping skills, and promotes adaptive responses to life's challenges.

Incorporating mental health support into the comprehensive care of seniors with fatty liver disease promotes holistic wellness, resilience, and improved quality of life. It's important for healthcare providers, caregivers, and loved ones to recognize the significance of mental health and offer appropriate resources and support to seniors as they navigate their health journey.

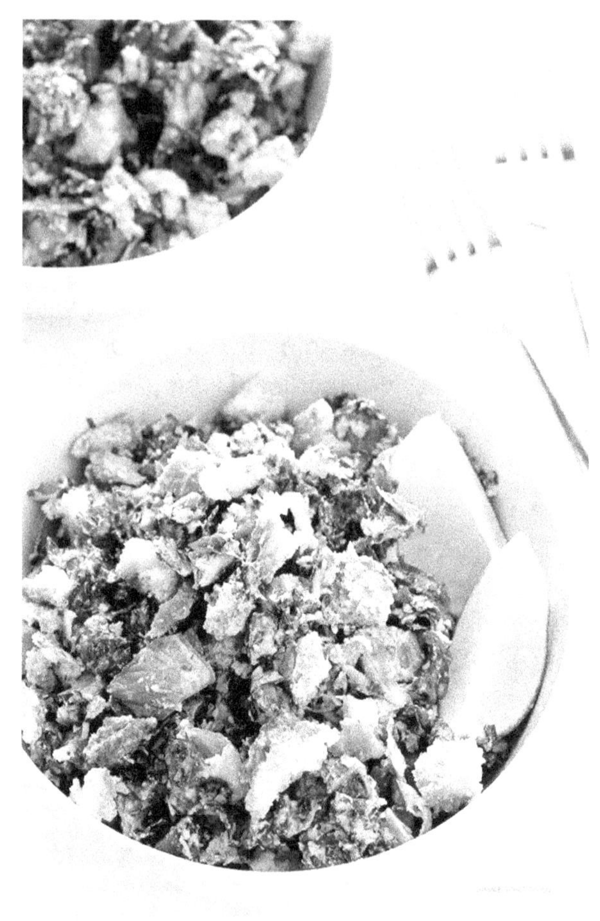

CHAPTER TEN

Long-Term Strategies for Maintaining Liver Health

Long-term maintenance of liver health is paramount for seniors managing fatty liver disease. In this final chapter, we'll explore strategies for sustaining liver health and preventing disease progression:

1. **Regular Monitoring and Follow-Up:**
   - Seniors should undergo regular check-ups and monitoring of liver function to assess disease progression and response to treatment.

   - Follow-up appointments with healthcare providers help track changes in liver enzymes, assess risk factors, and adjust treatment plans as needed.

2. **Consistent Adherence to Lifestyle Modifications:**
   - Consistency is key when it comes to implementing dietary changes, exercise routines, and stress management techniques.

   - Seniors should prioritise adherence to lifestyle modifications to maintain optimal liver health and prevent disease exacerbation.

3. **Ongoing Education and Support:**
   - Continued education about fatty liver disease and its management empowers seniors to make informed decisions about their health.

   - Support groups, online resources, and educational materials provide valuable information, encouragement, and camaraderie for individuals navigating fatty liver management.

4. **Stay Informed About Treatment Advances:**
   - Stay abreast of advancements in fatty liver treatment options, research findings, and emerging therapies.

   - Seniors should consult with their healthcare providers to explore new treatment modalities or clinical trials that may offer potential benefits for managing fatty liver disease.

5. **Holistic Approach to Wellness:**
   - Embrace a holistic approach to wellness that addresses physical, emotional, and spiritual aspects of health.

   - Seniors should prioritise self-care, meaningful connections, and activities that promote overall well-being and fulfilment.

By adopting these long-term strategies for maintaining liver health, seniors can optimise their quality of life, minimise disease complications, and enjoy a fulfilling and active lifestyle well into their golden years.

The completion of the chapters provides comprehensive guidance for seniors navigating the challenges of managing fatty liver disease. Each chapter offers valuable insights, practical tips, and actionable steps to support liver health, improve overall well-being, and enhance quality of life. As seniors implement these strategies into their daily lives, they empower themselves to take control of their health and embrace a future of vitality and wellness.

Monitoring Liver Function and Disease Progression

Monitoring liver function and disease progression is crucial for seniors with fatty liver disease to assess the effectiveness of treatment, detect complications early, and make necessary adjustments to their management plan. Here are key aspects of monitoring liver health:

Liver Function Tests:
   - Liver function tests, including alanine aminotransferase (ALT), aspartate aminotransferase (AST), gamma-glutamyl transferase (GGT), and alkaline phosphatase (ALP), are essential for assessing liver health and detecting abnormalities in liver enzymes.

Imaging Studies:

- Imaging studies such as ultrasound, computed tomography (CT), or magnetic resonance imaging (MRI) can provide detailed images of the liver, allowing healthcare providers to evaluate liver size, detect fatty deposits, and identify signs of inflammation or scarring.

Transient Elastography (FibroScan):

- Transient elastography, commonly known as FibroScan, is a non-invasive imaging technique used to assess liver stiffness and fibrosis (scarring). FibroScan provides valuable information about the severity of liver damage and helps guide treatment decisions.

Liver Biopsy:

- In some cases, a liver biopsy may be performed to obtain a tissue sample for microscopic examination. A liver biopsy helps determine the extent of liver damage, assess the degree of inflammation and fibrosis, and guide treatment recommendations.

Monitoring Metabolic Factors:

- Seniors with fatty liver disease often have metabolic risk factors such as obesity, diabetes, high cholesterol, and hypertension. Monitoring metabolic parameters, including blood glucose levels, lipid profile, and blood pressure, is essential for managing these comorbidities and reducing the risk of disease progression.

Assessment of Comorbidities:

- Seniors with fatty liver disease are at increased risk of developing complications such as cardiovascular disease, kidney disease, and certain cancers. Regular monitoring and management of comorbidities are essential for optimising overall health and reducing the risk of complications.

Evaluation of Lifestyle Factors:

- Assessing lifestyle factors such as diet, physical activity, alcohol consumption, and medication use is important for understanding their impact on liver health and disease progression. Healthcare providers can offer guidance and support to seniors in making healthy lifestyle choices.

Risk Stratification and Monitoring Frequency:

- Seniors with fatty liver disease may be stratified into different risk categories based on the severity of liver damage, presence of comorbidities, and other risk factors. The frequency of monitoring may vary based on individual risk profiles and treatment goals.

Patient Education and Empowerment:

- Educating seniors about the importance of monitoring liver function and disease progression empowers them to take an active role in their health care. Encouraging regular follow-up visits, adhering to recommended monitoring protocols, and reporting any new or worsening symptoms are key aspects of patient engagement.

Collaborative Care Approach:

- Monitoring liver function and disease progression requires a collaborative approach involving primary care providers, hepatologists, gastroenterologists, and other healthcare professionals. Communication and coordination among members of the healthcare team ensure comprehensive care and optimal outcomes for seniors with fatty liver disease.

Regular Follow-Up Visits:

- Seniors should schedule regular follow-up visits with their healthcare providers to assess liver function, review treatment efficacy, and address any concerns or questions. Follow-up visits allow for ongoing evaluation and adjustment of the management plan as needed.

Patient Advocacy and Support:

- Seniors should be encouraged to advocate for their own health care needs and seek support from healthcare providers, caregivers, and support groups. Open communication, shared decision-making, and access to resources promote effective disease management and improved quality of life.

By implementing a comprehensive approach to monitoring liver function and disease progression, seniors with fatty liver disease can receive timely interventions, optimise treatment outcomes, and maintain optimal liver health for the long term. Regular monitoring provides valuable insights into disease management and empowers seniors to take proactive steps toward improved health and well-being.

Holistic Approaches to Sustaining Liver Health Over Time

Maintaining liver health requires a holistic approach that addresses various aspects of physical, mental, and emotional well-being. Here are key holistic approaches seniors can adopt to sustain liver health over time:

1. Healthy Diet:
   - Eat a balanced diet rich in fruits, vegetables, whole grains, lean proteins, and healthy fats. Limit intake of processed foods, sugary beverages, saturated fats, and excess alcohol, all of which can contribute to liver damage.

2. Regular Physical Activity:
   - Engage in regular aerobic exercise, strength training, and flexibility exercises to promote overall fitness and support liver function. Aim for at least 150 minutes of moderate-intensity aerobic activity per week, as advised by health standards.

3. Maintain a Healthy Weight:

- Achieve and maintain a healthy weight through a combination of diet, exercise, and lifestyle modifications. Excess body weight, particularly abdominal obesity, is a significant risk factor for fatty liver disease and other liver conditions.

4. Manage Chronic Conditions:

- Effectively manage chronic conditions such as diabetes, high blood pressure, high cholesterol, and obesity, as they are closely linked to liver health. Adhering to treatment plans, monitoring symptoms, and making necessary lifestyle changes can help prevent complications and support liver function.

5. Limit Alcohol Consumption:

- Limit alcohol consumption or abstain from alcohol altogether, especially if diagnosed with liver disease or at risk of developing liver-related complications. Excessive alcohol intake can exacerbate liver damage and increase the risk of liver cirrhosis, fatty liver disease, and liver cancer.

6. Stay Hydrated:

- Drink an adequate amount of water throughout the day to support liver function and promote overall hydration. Proper hydration helps flush toxins from the body and supports various metabolic processes in the liver.

7. Practice Stress Management:

- Incorporate stress management techniques such as mindfulness meditation, deep breathing exercises, yoga, and relaxation techniques into daily routines. Chronic stress can contribute to liver inflammation and impair liver function over time.

8. Get Sufficient Sleep:

- Prioritise getting sufficient sleep each night to support overall health and well-being. Aim for 7-8 hours of quality sleep to allow the body to repair and regenerate tissues, including the liver.

9. Promote Mental and Emotional Well-being:

- Foster positive mental and emotional well-being through social connections, hobbies, relaxation activities, and meaningful relationships. Addressing mental health concerns and seeking support when needed contributes to overall wellness and resilience.

10. Regular Health Screenings:

- Schedule regular health screenings and check-ups with healthcare providers to monitor liver function, assess risk factors, and detect potential health concerns early. Early detection and intervention can prevent complications and improve treatment outcomes.

11. Educate Yourself:

- Stay informed about liver health, risk factors, symptoms of liver disease, and available treatment options. Knowledge empowers individuals to make informed decisions about their health and take proactive steps toward liver health.

12. Seek Support and Guidance:
   - Seek support from healthcare providers, registered dietitians, mental health professionals, and support groups specialising in liver health. Collaboration with healthcare professionals and peers provides valuable guidance, encouragement, and resources for sustaining liver health over time.

Adopting holistic approaches to liver health involves making lifestyle choices that prioritise overall well-being and support liver function. By incorporating these strategies into daily routines and maintaining consistency over time, seniors can promote liver health, reduce the risk of liver disease, and enjoy a higher quality of life in the long term.

CONCLUSION

In conclusion, the "Fatty Liver Diet Cookbook for Seniors" serves as a comprehensive resource for seniors navigating the complexities of fatty liver disease management. Throughout this guide, we have explored the fundamental principles of fatty liver disease, the importance of diet and nutrition, practical meal planning tips, and lifestyle modifications tailored specifically for seniors.

Managing fatty liver disease requires a multifaceted approach that encompasses dietary modifications, regular physical activity, stress management techniques, and ongoing monitoring of liver health. By adopting a liver-friendly diet rich in whole foods, incorporating superfoods, and making lifestyle changes that promote overall well-being, seniors can effectively manage fatty liver disease and improve their quality of life.

It is essential for seniors to prioritise their liver health by staying informed, proactive, and empowered in their journey towards wellness. By working closely with healthcare professionals, embracing healthy habits, and seeking support from loved ones, seniors can navigate the challenges of fatty liver disease with confidence and resilience.

As we conclude this journey, let us remember that optimal liver health is achievable through mindful choices, nourishing foods, and holistic lifestyle practices. With dedication, commitment, and a sense of empowerment, seniors can embrace a future of vitality, wellness, and longevity, ensuring that every day is lived to the fullest.